a
Healthier
YOU

The Pocket Guide
for Living A Happy &
Healthy Life At Any Age

DAVID L. VAUGHN

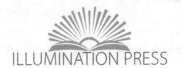
ILLUMINATION PRESS

ISBN: 978-1-7322384-0-4

Cover Design and Interior Layout by AugustPride, LLC

DEDICATION

This book is dedicated to Flois and Konrad Knolle, Joshua and Carolyn Simpkins, Clarence and Faye Hicks and to my Lifelong friend, Joan Harrison.

This book is also dedicated to those who have been putting their health on the back burner. The time is NOW for you to get flt and healthy so that you can live a longer and happier life.

To: Joyce
I hope you enjoy the book.
Best Wishes and God bless you!

David Vaughn
8/26/2018

CONTENTS

LIVE YOUR LIFE NOT YOUR AGE

Have you ever thought about getting older? Are they happy thoughts?

Most people dread getting older. They imagine an endless tirade of aches and pains, frequent visits to a myriad of doctors, and a daily regimen of medicines. The highlight of your day is your favorite daytime television show.

Getting older seems to be synonymous with slowing down. Instead of looking forward to your golden years with excitement, you might be dreading them. But getting older doesn't have to mean getting weaker. In fact, at 78, I have more activity, energy, and excitement in my life than people 20-30 years younger than I am.

What's Age Got To Do With It?
To me, 78 is just a number. It tells people how many years I've lived on this Earth, but that's it. My age does not define my mental or physical condition. And, it certainly does not define how I live my life. In fact, at 78, I enjoy a vibrant, active life that brings me lots of joy and fulfillment.

So a typical week for me will include 20 minutes of cardio and strength training a day, meetings with my special events and catering clients, Monday and Tuesday night choir rehearsals, volunteering with the local theatre group, Thursday dance classes, weekly night out with friends, playing tennis on Saturdays, and attending church services on Sunday.

My Kickstart to a Longer, Happier, & Healthier Life.

I have not always been this active or felt the way I do about things. It really happened when I was in my early 40's. One evening on my way home from work, I saw a woman on the side of the road with a flat tire. I was raised to be a gentleman so I stopped to see if I could be of assistance. As I approached, I saw that this woman was very beautiful. Her skin was so clear and radiant. At first she refused my offer of help.

"I got this," she said as she lifted the spare tire out of the trunk.

I insisted that she allow me to help and she finally agreed. As I changed the tire we engaged in small talk. Something she said intrigued me so I did something that most people would advise against—I asked her how old she was.

Instead of admonishing me, she immediately answered, "I am a proud 75!"

I was astonished. Her response intrigued me even more. This woman didn't look a day over 45. How had she stopped the aging process? What was her secret for looking and acting so young?

"Fish and fowl and things that grow," was her response.

Noticing the confused look on my face, she explained further," I only eat poultry, seafood, vegetables, and fruits." She went on to explain that she also stayed active and exercised every day.

After I met this lovely angel, I was inspired to change the way I was living. I was encouraged by the idea that I could change just a few things in my life and see such amazing results. But, I was also a bit apprehensive…

Give up bacon? No grilled cheese? Was that even possible?

I doubted that I could make the changes she recommended. But, then I looked down at my belly. I could barely see my feet. My bad eating and sedentary lifestyle had taken a drastic toll on my life. Here I was amazed at the vibrancy and vitality of a 75 year old woman and I, in my early 40's, was barely able to change a tire without getting winded. I knew I had to make changes now or I might not get to see 75.

I wish I could tell you my journey to ageless living

was easy. I wish I could tell you that as soon as you make the decision to adopt a healthier lifestyle everything around you changes and you are transformed immediately. But, I can't. When I started my journey, it was difficult at first. I had to not only change my eating habits; I also had to change my mindset. My journey wasn't perfect, but it was definitely worth it.

If I would have continued my life the way I was living at 45, the life I now live at 78 would never have been possible. I might have ended up frail with mental and physical challenges that could keep me bed-ridden or may even worse. Instead, however, I am fit in mind, body, and spirit.

I want the same for you.

First Things First
Before we go any further, I feel it necessary to address a few things…

First, in this pocket guide, I am sharing with you my recommendations for healthy eating and living. These recommendations are based on my personal experience and the experiences of others who live a similar lifestyle. I am not a doctor or medical expert. I strongly advise you to consult with your medical professional before making any drastic dietary changes.

Second, this is not a diet. I do not believe in diets because once you stop following a diet, you return to the same unhealthy habits you had before. That's why so many people experience the yo-yo effect of up and down weight loss and gain. This is a lifestyle change. My hope is that you will develop new eating habits that will last a lifetime.

Third, you must make the decision to stick with it. You don't have to be perfect, but you must be willing to persevere. Trust the process and know that every day you will.

And, last, but certainly not least…take it one step at a time. Do not try to do everything at once. It will seem tempting to try to incorporate all of the tips I share in this book at the same time. But, if you do that you'll quickly get overwhelmed and give up. Instead, take one key at a time. Master one concept then add the others gradually, one by one.

Now, if you are ready to begin your journey to ageless living.

Let's Go!

RULE 1
SAY YES TO YOU!

The first and most important shift you must make on your journey to ageless living is a mindset shift.

Throughout this book, I'll be sharing with you lots of things you will want to give up to improve your health and well-being. I will recommend several foods that you limit or cut out of your diet altogether.

For most people this is where the journey starts and ends. Just the thought of giving up a few unhealthy foods sends them into a tailspin. Never mind that the foods they want to so desperately hold on to are poisoning them and preventing them from living a long, healthy life. The only thing they are concerned with is being able to eat whatever they want. They say yes to the fatty, processed, and sugary foods and in turn they say no to themselves and the happy, healthy life they desire.

I don't want you to be like most people.
Instead of reading this book and thinking about the things that you'll be giving up, shift your focus to all the things you will be gaining. As you say no to the unhealthy lifestyle you've been living, you'll

in turn say yes to a happier, healthier life.

- ✓ **YES!** to a longer, healthier life!
- ✓ **YES!** to more energy and vitality!
- ✓ **YES!** to softer, more radiant, and glowing skin!
- ✓ **YES!** to better fitting clothes in a smaller size!
- ✓ **YES!** to reducing my risk for heart disease, obesity, and diabetes!
- ✓ **YES!** to a healthy brain and a more focused mind!
- ✓ **YES!** to a fit, firm body with fluid joints and limbs!
- ✓ **YES!** to less stress and better sleep!

As you are reading this book and you come to a section that makes you cringe and say, this is too much for me to do, come back to this section.

Remind yourself of all you have to gain if you stick it out.

Now, before you go any further, make a list of all the things you will be able to say yes to when you say no to an unhealthy lifestyle. You can use the list above as a guide, but I invite you to make your list unique to you.

I'M SAYING YES TO ME!

Use this space to make a list of all the things you want to say yes to as you begin to live a healthier life.

_____

_____

_____

_____

_____

_____

_____

_____

_____

_____

_____

_____

_____

_____

_____

_____

_____

_____

_____

RULE 2
FORGET WHITES. THINK COLORS.

The world of food has an amazing array of colors—reds, yellows, purples, greens, blues and oranges. The entire rainbow is available to us and every day we have the wonderful opportunity to taste that rainbow.

When you eat a diet mainly comprised of white foods you miss out on the essential key ingredients you need to live a healthy life. What's more—white, starchy foods take you over your blood sugar limits and they can cause you to have less energy and lots of trouble focusing and concentrating.

So why are colors so important? Take a look at the list below to see some of the health benefits from foods of different colors.

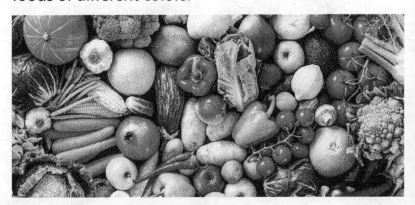

Red/Purple/Blue

Beets Kidney Beans	Iron, fiber, and folic acid for heart health and memory function. (The beans have lots of protein, too)
Blueberries Cranberries Raspberries Strawberries Grapefruit Red Bell Peppers	Vitamin C and Vitamin A for excellent eye and skin health
Eggplant Prunes	Fiber for staying fuller longer and great digestive health
Cherries Figs Tomatoes	Potassium to lower blood pressure

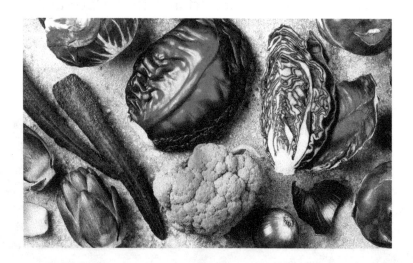

Oranges/Yellows

Cantaloupe Carrots Corn Oranges Orange/Yellow Bell Pepper Papaya Peaches Mango Squash Sweet Potatoes	Folic Acid, Vitamin C, potassium, and bromelane to lower blood pressure, reduce swelling, and infection.

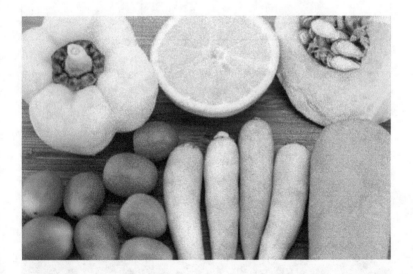

Greens

Apples Asparagus Avocado Broccoli Brussel Sprouts Cabbage Celery Cucumber Grapes Green Beans Green Peppers	Guava Herbs (basil, thyme, cilantro, parsley) Honey Dew Melon Kale Kiwis Pears Peas Spinach Zucchini	Fiber, Vitamin A, Vitamin C, folic acid to reduce risk of cancer, prevent heart disease, strengthen bones and teeth, and boost immune system.

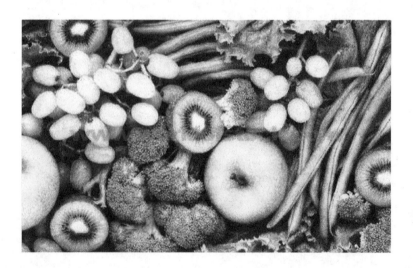

I shared with you the large variety of colorful foods and their benefits because I wanted to show you the abundance of foods you can eat before I started to tell you about the foods I recommend you take out of your diet.

When I first started on my journey to a healthier lifestyle, this was the toughest part. Most of the foods I was eating were filled with white flours and sugars. These foods were so tasty to me because they were highly processed with lots of additives that made them taste great. And, although they tasted really (really really) good, they were not so good for my health. My large protruding belly and non-visible toes were the proof of that.

So I made the decision to strictly limit and reduce the amount of white foods I eat. I highly recommend you do the same.

This means reducing and cutting out foods like

• Pancakes • Waffles	• White Bread • Cakes • Pies	• Cereal • White rice

I know you are probably looking at that list and saying oh no! I can't possibly cut out those foods. But, I ask you to remember Rule #1—Say yes to YOU!

The foods I mentioned above are just a few of the foods that you want to stay away from. In general you want to avoid any foods that are highly processed and contain large amounts of white flour, sugar, and salt.

With all the processing and additives these foods are very tasty yet they are not very satisfying. That's why you can eat them in large quantities and still feel hungry. In other words you have to eat more of these foods more often to feel full. All of this leads to a higher calorie intake and in turn, leads to uncontrollable weight gain.

Put This Rule Into Action
Try an experiment to see just what forgetting the whites can do for you. For sixty days, restrict your intake of white foods with refined flours and sugars. Instead of white rice and pasta, use brown rice and whole wheat pasta. Switch white breads for rye, pumpernickel, and barley breads. Reduce or eliminate processed foods like cookies, pies, cakes. Try these changes for sixty days and take note of the health and energy you will experience.

60 DAY NO WHITES CHALLENGE

In the space provided with how you are feeling on that day

DAY 1	DAY 2	DAY 3	DAY 4	DAY 5
DAY 6	DAY 7	DAY 8	DAY 9	DAY 10
DAY 11	DAY 12	DAY 13	DAY 14	DAY 15
DAY 16	DAY 17	DAY 18	DAY 19	DAY 20
DAY 21	DAY 22	DAY 23	DAY 24	DAY 25
DAY 26	DAY 27	DAY 28	DAY29	DAY 30

60 DAY NO WHITES CHALLENGE

DAY 31	DAY 32	DAY 33	DAY 34	DAY 35
DAY 36	DAY 37	DAY 38	DAY 39	DAY 40
DAY 41	DAY 42	DAY 43	DAY 44	DAY 45
DAY 46	DAY 47	DAY 48	DAY 49	DAY 50
DAY 51	DAY 52	DAY 53	DAY 54	DAY 55
DAY 56	DAY 57	DAY 58	DAY59	DAY 60

RULE 3
READ THE LABELS

It is essential that you read all packages and cans. One of the main reasons you might be struggling to see changes in your body even when you think you are eating healthy is because you have no idea what you are really eating. A lot of the foods most people think are healthy actually contain additives and ingredients that do more harm than good.

Juice is a primary example. Many fruit juices have less than 40% of real fruit juice. That's right, the next time you grab some cranberry juice, look to see how much is juice and how much is water. See also if it contains fructose or corn syrup or other sweeteners.

In fact, you should read all of your labels so you can see what you are getting. This will be very educational!

Here's what to look for on your food labels:

First, take a look at the big picture. Scan the food label to check for calories, sodium, fat, protein, carbohydrates, vitamins, and nutrients. When you scan the label you will be able to see how this food fits within your overall health goals. I can remember how surprised I was when I saw how many calories and fat grams were actually in some of the health bars I was eating—no wonder I wasn't losing any weight!

Next, take a look at the serving size. Many times we eat way more of a food than we should. Take chips for instance. The typical serving size for chips is 1 ounce or about 15 chips. Each serving size is approximately 160 calories. But, when was the last time you only ate 16 chips? Probably never. Most people eat 3 – 4 servings of chips in a single setting which means they are eating 480 – 600 calories. This doesn't' include the amount of fat, carbohydrates, and sodium you are consuming. That's why it's important to really understand the true serving size measure.

Finally, look at the list of ingredients. I recommend not eating foods with ingredients you cannot pronounce. The FDA requires all food labels to list every single ingredient and additive included in a food item. The ingredients most prevalent in your food are listed first. If you see sugars, salts, carbohydrates listed before proteins, vitamins, and minerals, you want to avoid those foods.

Try It Out
For the fun of it, stop by a store, pick up a box of plain breadcrumbs and read the label. You will be

surprised as to what they put into breadcrumbs, called plain breadcrumbs. The flavored ones have a list of ingredients as long as the container itself.

Take It A Step Further
Eat Fresh!

If you are thinking that canned and packaged foods aren't so bad—think again.

Not only do most canned and packaged foods go through lots of processing, the cans and packages themselves can contain dangerous chemicals.

For the best health benefits, I recommend you severely restrict the packaged and canned foods. Foods that have been processed for canning and packaging have been altered and their nutritional state has been compromised.

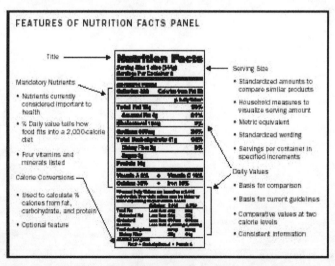

RULE 4
WATER IS LIFE

I know you've heard it many times before. Drinking water is essential to your health. Most experts recommend that you drink at least sixty four ounces or eight glasses of water every day. I agree.

Over the past three decades of my life I've found that drinking more water has caused me to have several amazing health benefits.

First, drinking more water energized my muscles. I found that it was much easier for me not just to workout but to work out for longer periods of time. The more water I drank the more fluid my movements became. I was able—and still am able—to do exercises that I wasn't even able to do in my twenties and thirties.

In addition to being more flexible with stronger muscles, I also found that my attitude shifted. I don't like to admit it but I was not so nice to be around before I started on my healthier lifestyle. I was often cranky. After doing some research I now know that I was cranky because my body was dehydrated. There is research that shows lack of adequate water intake can affect your mood and cause you to be grumpy.

On top of those great benefits - I lost lots of weight, too!

I found out that I was eating way too much. It's true that sometimes when we think we are hungry, we are actually thirsty. As I started to drink more water I found that my food cravings lessened. I also found that when I drank a glass of water before a meal, I ate less and I felt more satisfied, much longer.

As I started seeing the tremendous benefits of drinking more water, I began to eliminate the sodas and other sugary drinks from my diet.

But, here's the thing…

When I started on my healthy journey, I mostly drank sodas and other sugary beverages. It was not unusual for me to consume two or three sodas in a day. When I changed my eating habits, I switched from sodas to bottled juices. But, that wasn't much better. Remember Rule #3, Read The Labels? Well, if you look at the contents of most juices you will see that their top ingredient is sugar. In some cases, drinking the juice was worse than drinking a soda.

Making the switch from sodas to juices and then to water was not easy for me and it definitely didn't happen overnight. It was a gradual process.

The first thing I had to do was to get over my addiction to sugary drinks. Yes, I said addiction. Most people don't realize it but they are actually addicted to sodas and sugary drinks. They say, "I like sodas but I could give them up at any time if I wanted…I just don't want to."

Have you ever thought something like that? If so, I have to tell you—the first step to overcoming an addiction is to admit you have one.

The next step is to make a decision to change. Remember, you are saying YES to a longer, healthier life.

One thing I will tell you is that cutting the sodas and sugary drinks out of your diet is a process you should take slowly. Most people try to go cold turkey and end up binging because they feel deprived. Don't try to shock your body by eliminating the sodas and sugary drinks all at once. If you do that your body will rebel against you and it will be almost impossible to make the switch on a long term basis. You must ease your body into the change gradually.

Here are some ways I've found to make drinking more water a lot easier.

Add flavor to your water.
Now you should know by now I'm not talking

about those powdery packets stores sell to add to your water. What I suggest is add fresh fruits to your water. Fill a pitcher with water and add strawberries, oranges, lemons, or maybe even grapefruit. You could also try adding herbs like mint, basil or lavender. Some veggies like cucumber or celery can also add a refreshing taste to your water.

You can even try some different combinations to add some variety. A few of my favorites are:

- Strawberry + Blueberry
- Watermelon + Rosemary
- Lemon + Lime + Grapefruit
- Apple + Cinnamon Sticks
- Mango + Pineapple

Dilute sugary drinks with water and ice.
If you have a long set in habit of drinking sodas, juices, lemonade, and sweet tea on a daily basis you can ease your way out of that habit by diluting your beverages with water.

To start you may fill your glass halfway with ice and then fill it three fourths of the way with the soda or juice, then fill it the rest of the way with water. Over time, you can add more ice, less soda, and more water. The change will be gradual and before long you'll have the entire glass filled with water, ice, and no soda.

Eat water rich foods.
One sneaky way to get your body to crave more water is to eat foods with a high water content. The more water you put into your body the more water your body will want. The next time you go to the grocery store, add fruits and vegetables that are high in water content to your shopping list.

Some top picks include:
- cucumber - 96% water
- zucchini - 95% water
- watermelon - 92% water
- grapefruit - 91% water
- radishes – 95% water
- lettuce – 95% water
- celery – 95% water
- tomatoes – 94% water
- green peppers – 93% water
- cauliflower – 92% water

Because of their high water content, a lot of these foods are considered to be negative calorie foods. This means that it takes more calories to digest these foods than they contain. You can eat as many of these foods as you like and not worry about gaining extra weight. In fact, you'll lose weight!

Stick With It!
The best advice I can give you for drinking more water is to stick with it. You don't have to be perfect and only drink water for the rest of your life. You can drink sodas and sugary drinks from time to time in limited quantities. Just focus on drinking more water than anything else.

Remember, this is a lifetime journey!

RULE 5
KNOW WHAT TO AVOID

We have talked a lot so far about what to add to your healthy eating lifestyle. Now, it's time to talk about what to avoid.

Before you go further, remind yourself of Rule #1. You might find yourself cringing at some of the suggestions I am about to make and be tempted to throw in the towel before you even begin. Don't give into that temptation. Also, remember, as with everything else in this book - take it one step at a time. So, with those recommendations in mind, here are a few suggestions of the foods you should avoid to help you live a happier and healthier life.

Avoid adding meat to season your vegetables. In the South, it's a common tradition to flavor vegetables with meat. I encourage you to eat lots of vegetables but, don't want you to destroy their nutritional value by adding meat when you cook them. Instead use natural seasonings.

For instance, when cooking green beans or collard greens, use onions, garlic, leeks, cilantro, basil, thyme, green peppers, red peppers, and celery. Anything but meat. No pork or red blood meat and no animal skin. No bacon, bacon fat, chicken skin, pork rind or pig's feet. In fact, just leave the pig alone.

Avoid beef, pork, and dark meat poultry.
Overall, beef, pork, and dark meat poultry are higher in fats and cholesterol. Although some of the leaner cuts can have less fat and cholesterol, they are never as low as white meat poultry or fish.

Avoid fried foods.
Frying foods - even vegetables - alter their quality and increase their calorie content. These foods are so packed in high concentrations of trans fats and that contribute to diseases like heart disease, cancer, diabetes, and hypertension.   If you must, use olive oil only. One tablespoon of olive oil with onions, peppers, carrots and chopped celery will give you enough oil base to stir-fry anything.

Forget the gravy.
Do you know how gravy is made? Grease, flour, water … Bad for you! Use the natural juices from your vegetables and poultry as your gravy.

Cut the Chocolate.
Some of you might be ready to throw this book away right now. No chocolate? For some that's like saying no air. Before you write me off altogether, let me say this—chocolate is not inherently bad. There are some benefits of pure

chocolate like antioxidants that can boost health. However, most people don't eat pure chocolate. The chocolate most people eat is combined with lots of fats and sugars. Not to mention, chocolate is high in the wrong kinds of caffeine.

Avoid Dairy.
One of the hardest for you to give up on is dairy— that's why I put this last. We are the only animals that continually drink milk after our nursing years. Yet we think we need it for the calcium and potassium. Well, you will find out that many of the fruits and vegetables we have discussed in this book contain all the calcium and potassium you will need. If you find you need more, use a calcium vitamin to supplement what you think you are missing.

Dairy does not just mean milk—dairy also includes butter, ice cream, yogurt, and cheese. For a long time many experts have been telling us to drink and eat more dairy to benefit our bodies. But, evidence has shown that these studies were mostly by scientists working for the dairy industry. More recent independent studies reveal that dairy could in fact lead to bone loss.

Sure, I like ice cream and cheese as much as the next person, but I willingly sacrifice them for my health. Before we head into the next rule for healthy living, I want to give you a few more things to avoid.

Avoid Going Along With The Crowd.

You must discuss this diet with your life partner or family if you do not live alone. You may have to cook your meals separately if your diet does not suit someone else. When you go out to eat with your family or friends, you may have to choose carefully from the menu and ask how things are prepared before you order them. It is hard to find food that does not include cheese as an ingredient. Also, when you are visiting friends or family on events, or holidays, you may have to take your personally prepared food with you or take something you can eat with you to prepare there. Don't worry about offending anybody when your health is concerned. Just insist on eating what you must and not what they fix. This is tough, but a must.

Avoid Getting Sidetracked.

Don't even think about getting off the plan because you have not had fried chicken or a bacon cheeseburger in a while. You don't need them and don't pamper yourself with the wrong foods.

I have heard many people say, "Well, I've been good and I haven't had a brownie or chocolate cake or ice cream. So, I'm just going to treat myself a bit." Feeding yourself unhealthy foods is not a treat. All can be lost if you adopt this attitude. Give it all up for at least three months so you can know the difference in your new non-toxic body. It can be hard, but you don't have to do it alone. Please get in touch with me if you need encouragement or have questions about any of the suggestions I've made in this book.

RULE 6
GET MOVING

All this discipline in eating becomes even more important when you add exercise to your lifestyle. It is just as important to wake your cells up and to move the rusty parts of your body as it is to nourish your body with good eating.

This is not difficult either. You just need to incorporate movement into your day. I mean simple exercise. If you can't bend over and touch your toes, for instance, you can at least try to reach for the ceiling. Yes, how many times a day do you stand on your toes and stretch your body to the sky?

In this section, I am going to share with you exercises that are simple and important to the rejuvenation of your body. You'll be reenergized, refreshed, and reinvigorated.

You don't need to have a huge budget to get more exercise. Gyms and fitness centers are good, but if their price is out of your range there are other options for adding more movement into your daily life. For instance, there is the lawn mower and vacuum cleaner that can help you work up a sweat as good as the rowing machine at your local fitness club. A walk around the block works just as well—and I think even better—than a walk on the treadmill.

Take a look at these sample exercises you can easily incorporate into your life without any cost at all.

Stretch it Out
Stretch to the sky on your toes, rising up and down at least12 times with your fingers reaching up. You will feel the pull inside your calves, shoulder blades, ankles, and butt. If you ever owned a pet (dog or cat), you will notice that they stretch as soon as they wake up. There must be something instinctive and right about stretching, and we need to know that also.

Balancing Act
Clasp both of your hands in the back with your arms outstretched and raise your hands as far as you can. Then pull your left arm as far as you can with your right hand and your right arm as far as you can with your left hand stretching from side to side. Bring them back to the center of your back and raise both arms with your hands clasped as far as you can. Do this simple exercise for at least three minutes.

Wings
Raise both hands and clasp them at the back of the neck. Bring your elbows together in the front

trying to touch them without letting your hands go. Open and close your elbows in the front as many as 20 times trying to touch them. You may be inches apart now, but after steady attempts, you will close the gap in two to three weeks.

Knee Bends

With feet flat on the floor, hold your hands outstretched in front of you and do as many as 15 knees bend as though you were sitting on a chair and do not lean forward. Of course, if you lean backward, you will land on your behind.

Knee Lifts

Standing tall, raise your knees to your chest, for a count of 10 per knee, as high as you can. Alternating, of course, unless you can bring them both up at the same time, (No way unless you are jumping).

Stretching has been the predominant exercise suggested so far, now on to the moving exercises. Whether you want to admit it to your body, or not, you need to increase the efficient intake of oxygen to your body. This activity is significant to increase the flow of oxygen to your blood. This increase will make the difference in your output of energy, mental capacity, intuition, patience and level of stress.

That was a nice way of saying you got to do some

physical exercise like running, walking, jumping or aerobics. I am not going to spend a lot of time on this subject. It is quite simple. You have to make the supreme sacrifice and put exercise in your program.

If you are too tired in the evening, get up earlier in the morning. If you can't fit it in the morning hours, put it in during the day, during your lunch hour or during the evening after work and before dinner. I even have friends who do their exercise before they go to bed.   For me, I can't do that way because the level of energy is too high for me to fall asleep. But this proves that people are different. So whatever your choice of exercise program, the important thing is to do it and not to fake it. Do it at least three times a week.

Stretch every day, but do movement every other day or three times a week. In the beginning, you will feel tight, and muscles will want to harden on you, but after a while, you will relax into the habit. Hopefully! There are several suggestions you should try.

Running in place for a short time is an easy way to get started. You can also try things like side-straddle hops; jump with a rope like a boxer; run around your house, your block, and your nearest athletic field; up and down flights of steps.

The purpose is to increase your heartbeat, stimulate the body's hormonal system and even to generate some sweat.

You can even "adopt a sport." Take up racquetball, tennis, biking, jogging, rollerblading; ice skating, bowling, aerobics and even dancing. Be very certain about which one; be diligent in the understanding of the sport; follow the ins and outs of the sport; know who is doing well with it, their names, their levels of achievement and what it will take for you to be serious about your game.

All I am trying to say is that exercise is necessary and should not be looked at as a major chore, but as a fun activity and you should want to do it. We are people who procrastinate too much. We let excuses get in the way of reality and productivity.

Exercise is a major part of keeping healthy. The more we do, the better we are. It is your body, and no one else can do it for you.

RULE 7
CONNECT YOUR MIND, BODY & SPIRIT

Living a longer, happier, and healthier life is more than just about what you eat and the exercises you do. Living a longer life will mean nothing if you are miserable in the process.

Life is to be enjoyed! Today we do not only have to care about our physical, financial and mental health, but most important is our spiritual health because what's happening on the inside of you will always show up on the outside.

Smiling instead of frowning, forgiving instead of blaming, forgetting instead of languishing, and loving instead of hating, and understand that what helps you to do all these things is at the heart of your spiritual health.

If your spirit is not forgiving, caring and loving, then you will not know the real meaning of life.

For those of us who are raised in the understanding and training of the Lord and Savior, Jesus Christ, it is the knowledge that keeps our faith alive. However, to know the way, to seek the answers and not to follow the teaching is also stressful.

Develop Your Faith

I have heard others say that they believe, but when it is time to demonstrate that belief, they spend hundreds of dollars on the lottery, palm readers and analysis instead of putting their faith to test. Faith is the key to understanding the mysteries of life. Even control freaks have to admit that God delivers when they can't. What they also had to learn was that when they put their trust in God and when they put their problems in God's hands, they had to leave them to God for Him to work them out.

I have heard others say it, but continue to do their piddling part to make things change, and they never do.

That means we can put worry to rest. Pray, save, trust, have faith, but don't worry about a thing. If it is meant to happen, it will. If not, then let it be. Worry only brings wrinkles, frowns, stomachaches and other ills. Faith and trust and thoughtful undertakings with hope, not worry can make the difference.

Release Your Financial Burdens

You might be wondering why I'm including this in a book about healthy living. But, you would be surprised how our financial health can affect our physical well- being. Stress over money concerns often leads to over eating and other unhealthy behaviors.

It is amazing how much stress we bring to ourselves. We spend too much time worrying about money matters when we should simply try to exercise discipline in the spending of money. It is amazing how many of us spend the same dollar more than once. Once it is paid out, it does not automatically appear back in our bank accounts or back into our pockets.

Spontaneous spending and shopping should be discontinued until you have the shopping money that is not already promised or due to go to somewhere else. It is also amazing how many of us say we are going to save for something and we never do. In fact, when you had the extra money, did you save it? When things were more abundant, did you put it aside for shopping and a rainy day? You know you didn't.

Learn to Love You
You must learn to feel good about yourself. You must learn to trust yourself, be proud of your accomplishments and treat yourself right.
First of all, you must take the attitude that you are the best in whatever you do. Teacher, bus

driver, janitor, nurse, singer—it doesn't matter your profession. What matters is that we carry a positive attitude with us and strive to be the best in our chosen profession, married or single, parent or not. Don't burden yourself with so many judgmental issues.

I remember hearing the famous Reverend Leon Sullivan saying that you can turn your stumbling blocks into stepping stones and your problems into opportunities.

Practice Gratitude

There will always be things in your life that aren't going exactly as you would like them to go—that's called life.

The reason why so many people find it difficult to change their unhealthy lifestyles is because they are focusing all of their attention on all the things that are preventing them from moving forward and neglecting to consider all of the things that will support them in their decision.

They look at how much they hate their job and the fact that they haven't gotten the promotion they want so they pick up the chocolate cake and sit on the couch binge watching television. But, if instead these same people looked at the fact that the job they have is keeping a roof over their heads and clothes on their back, they might have a reason to be grateful. The pity part would end and they would be more likely to engage in healthier activities.

Even in the toughest of circumstances there are things for which you can be grateful. As you increase in gratitude you will have a more positive attitude. That positive attitude will bring you more hope and in turn, that hope will give you more incentive to want to live a longer and healthier life.

Reframe Your Problems
Somehow the will and the way have always been there. Use your situation to do better, look at the positive side of it. Use it as your stepping stone to a better position or a better job within the organization or out of the organization. Look at your problems as opportunities for change. See what is at the heart of the problem; seize the opportunity to solve your problem, instead of complaining about it.

Once you adopt a positive attitude, stop complaining and make the best of your time on this earth, you will be a healthier you. When asked how you are feeling, always say "great," joyful," "wonderful," "terrific," or "truly blessed." People

will do a double take and say "really." They might
even ask you how come? This will give you an
opportunity to witness to your personal blessing
and to share the new you, the positive you and
the healthier you.

SUGGESTED FOOD LIST

Here is a listing of the food you should incorporate in your healthy selections for a better health.

Breakfast:
- Oatmeal
- Grits (without milk)
- Eggs
- Apples (sliced and sautéed with cinnamon
- Salmon cakes
- Turkey sausage (remove the skin which is made of pig intestines)
- Raisin Bread
- Pumpernickel toast
- Rye toast

Vegetables:
- Carrots (Honey, cinnamon & ginger)
- Broccoli
- Zucchini/Squash (onions, vegetable stock. Bread crumbs topping)
- Cauliflower
- Spinach
- Kale
- Collard Greens (Use smoked Turkey instead of Pork) Or Onions and garlic salt.
- Turnip greens
- Green Beans

- Black eye peas
- Black Beans
- Pinto Beans
- Cannelli Beans
- Garbanzo (Chick Peas)
- Navy/white Beans
- Lima Beans
- (spice your vegetables up with fresh chopped Red Peppers, Green Peppers, Onions, Cilantro, Green Onions, Bay leaves, Thyme)

Starches:
- Brown rice
- Rice a Roni with black rice
- Sweet Potatoes/yams
- Golden potatoes
- Cous cous
- Flavored Pasta (Other than white)

Meats:
- Chicken, Baked, with Ginger Ale and garlic; baked and smothered with Rosemary
- Turkey, Duck,
- Salmon, Other fish
- Shrimp, Crab, Lobster
- Mussels
- Clams

Fruit:
All fruit   (at least 3 servings a day)

SAMPLE MEAL SELECTIONS

1
Roasted Turkey with gravy Sautéed Green Beans
Mashed Potatoes Cranberry/apple sauce

2
Cajun Baked fish
Red Cabbage & Rice

3
Baked chicken breast in ginger ale and garlic
Baked Zucchini/squash

4
Roasted Salmon in honey/lime sauce
baked potatoes
Spinach

5
Seafood Medley with Shrimp, salmon and diced tomatoes served over rice or pasta
Collard/ turnip or kale

6
Pulled BBQ Turkey Drumstick
Sweet Potato soufflé
Black eyed peas

7
Chicken fingers in Rosemary Gravy
Pinto Beans
French Fried Cauliflower

8
Stir fried Shrimp & Vegetables
Bowtie Pasta

9
Maryland Crab Cakes
Green Peas
Golden Mashed Potatoes

RECIPES FOR
SAMPLE MEAL SELECTIONS

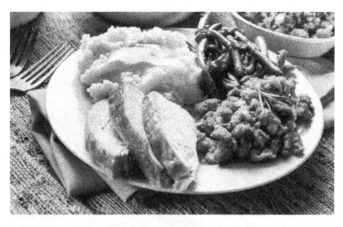

ROASTED TURKEY WITH GRAVY/ GREEN BEANS AND MASHED POTATOES

Ingredients:
1 full Turkey Breast
½ teaspoon salt
½ teaspoon ground pepper
Place in oven and bake for 30 minutes at 350 degrees

....
3 cups green beans
½ cup of chopped onions
½ teaspoon of salt & pepper
1 teaspoon of soy sauce
½ cup water
Place onions and 3 tablespoons of olive oil in pan or pot and stir for 3 minutes.
Add green beans, water and spices and stir for

another 3 minutes. Turn off and add soy sauce.
Ready to serve.

....

3 medium size potatoes
1 teaspoon salt
½ teaspoon white pepper
1 tablespoon margarine
1 teaspoon of garlic powder

Preparation:

1. Peel and dice potatoes and boil for 8 minutes or until potatoes are soft.
2. Mash potatoes and add seasoning
3. Top with juices from Roasted turkey for gravy

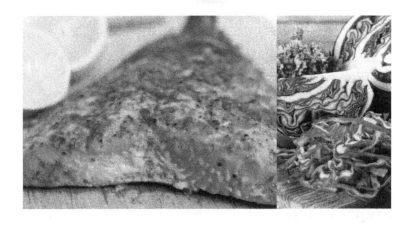

CAJUN BAKED FISH/RED CABBAGE & RICE

(For Fish) Ingredients:

There are so many different fish available. I recommend the fish you can purchase as fillet and with fewer bones:

Ocean Perch	Flounder	Mahi Mahi
Grouper	Halibut	Orange Roughy
Tilapia	Catfish	Snapper
Cod	Whiting	Trout

3 or 4 pieces of fish of your choice
1 teaspoon of Cajun Seasoning or a pinch of paprika, cayenne, turmeric & white pepper
½ teaspoon of salt

Preparation:

Place fish on baking dish and dry rub the fish with

the seasoning. Bake for 10 – 12 minutes at 350º.

(For Cabbage and Rice) Ingredients:

½ Head of red cabbage sliced, ½ of cabbage chopped

1 Sweet green pepper and/ or red pepper sliced

1 Onion ½ sliced & ½ chopped

1 cup of rice

3 cups of water or vegetable broth

1 teaspoon of salt and pepper

1 teaspoon of Cayenne pepper

1 tablespoon of cumin

Preparation:

1. Put cabbage, pepper and onion in skillet and stir fry with ½ cup of olive, vegetable or canola oil.
2. Stir until they all start to soften and absorb the oil. And add the spices while stirring.
3. Then add 1 cup of water or vegetable broth. Continue to stir and add the rest of the water or broth.
4. Bring to a boil and add the cup of rice stir one last time then cover and let it simmer for 5 minutes.
5. Put on low and let it simmer for 5 more minutes.
6. Turn off the heat and let stand for ten minutes without opening the top.

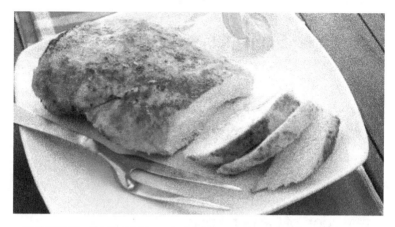

BAKED CHICKEN BREAST IN GINGER ALE AND GARLIC/ BAKED ZUCCHINI/SQUASH

(For Chicken) Ingredients:

3 or 4 chicken breast boneless (one for each diner)
½ teaspoon salt and pepper,
2 tablespoons of corn starch
1 tablespoon of ground ginger
1 tablespoon of garlic powder
1 glass of ginger ale

Preparation:

1. Place chicken breast in baking dish or pan (choose one with a matching top)
2. Sprinkle spices and corn starch on chicken and bake for 10 minutes uncovered
3. remove and pour ginger ale over all the chicken and cover and bake for 40 minutes.

4. (p.s.) do not remove cover until it is time to serve. Pour the juice over each breast as it is being plated. Also, this recipe can be used for any part of chicken with or without bones.

(For Squash) Ingredients:
4 to 6 medium size squash. (sliced to ¼ inch)
2 medium size or 1 large onion (sliced to 1/8 inch) round or half round
I cup of Italian bread crumbs.

Preparation:
1. Choose a baking dish with a top
2. Layer 1 layer of squash with 1 layer of onions then sprinkle bread crumbs
3. Do this three or four times or until you have no more to layer. Top off with the balance
4. of bread crumb and sprinkle a touch of olive oil over the entire casserole Bake at 350 for 40 minutes.

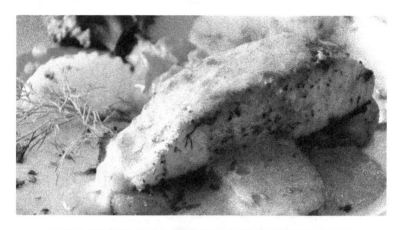

ROASTED SALMON IN HONEY-LIME SAUCE/ BAKED POTATO AND SPINACH

(For Salmon) Ingredients:

3 to 4 slices of Salmon (one for each diner)
½ teaspoon of salt and pepper
2 tablespoons of Honey and 2 tablespoons of fresh lime juice (mix together)

Preparation:

1. Preheat oven to 350 degrees. Place salmon on oven tray and sprinkle salt and pepper on ·each piece.
2. Spread honey -lime mixture on the top of each piece and bake for15 minutes

(For Potato) Ingredients:

Select 1 potato per person. Rinse clean and place on oven shelf

Preparation:
1. Bake potatoes in oven 30 minutes prior to putting the salmon in the oven.
2. In 45 minutes both should be done at the same time. (if using aluminum foil, allow ten more minutes for baking.)

(For Spinach) Ingredients:
2 cans of spinach or 2 bunches of fresh spinach (Cut the stems off).
½ teaspoon of salt and pepper
¼ cup of water
1 hard-boiled egg

Preparation:
1. Wash and clean fresh spinach or drain and rinse canned spinach in colander.
2. Put spinach in a quart pan and add ¼ cup of water, salt and pepper, stir and simmer for a few minutes until the spinach heats up and the fresh spinach gets soft. In the meantime, boil one egg for garnish on spinach.
3. Slice egg for garnish on spinach and sprinkle salt and pepper to taste.

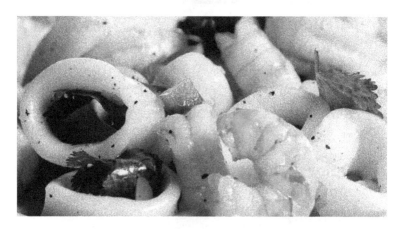

SEAFOOD MEDLEY WITH SHRIMP, SALMON AND DICED TOMATOES/RICE OR PASTA/FRESH GREENS

(For Seafood) Ingredients:

2 cups of cleaned, tail off shrimp
2 cups of canned or fresh salmon
1 28 ounce can of diced tomatoes
(if desired, other seafood can be added, i.e. clams, mussels, scallops, lobster)
1 teaspoon of salt and pepper,
1 tablespoon of Old Bay Seasoning
1 green pepper/onion chopped
1 bay leaf
l/2 cup of chopped parsley or cilantro

Preparation:

1. In 2-3 quart pan place tomatoes and all items

except seafood in the pot and stir until a simmer begins.

2. Add seafood and simmer for 5 minutes. Select an oven type bowl or pan with cover and bake for 20 minutes at 350 temperature. Serve over rice or favorite pasta

3. Serve with Collards, Turnip or Kale as a green accent to the dish. These can be freshly made or frozen or canned greens. Simply cook to taste adding salt and pepper.

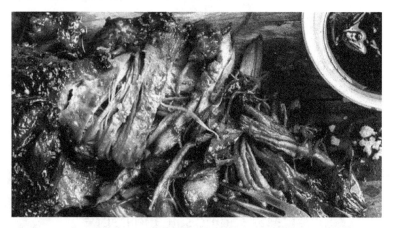

PULLED BBQ TURKEY DRUMSTICK, SWEET POTATO SOUFFLÉ AND BLACK EYED PEAS

(For Turkey) Ingredients:

4 turkey drumsticks
1 teaspoon salt and ground pepper
5 cups of water in sauce pan
½ cup of BBQ sauce (during cooking.)
1 cup of BBQ Sauce (for after cooking)

Preparation:

1. Boil the above together for 30 minutes. Let cool for 10 minutes. Pull meat off turkey bone.
2. Add cup of BBQ sauce to Turkey (your choice for thickness) Similar to Pulled Pork

(For Sweet Potato) Ingredients:

4 medium sized sweet potatoes or 3 yams

½ teaspoon of nutmeg
½ teaspoon of nutmeg
½ teaspoon of grated or fresh ginger
2 tablespoons of margarine

Preparation:
1. Boil potatoes/yams unpeeled until fork penetrates with ease.
2. Peal and mash and add spices and margarine
3. Bake for 20 minutes or eat as is.

(For Black Eye Peas) Ingredients:
2 cups of black eye peas
4 cups water
1/2 teaspoon of salt / pepper
¼ cup of chopped onions
½ teaspoon of garlic powder

Preparation:
1. Bring to a boil and let boil for 10 minutes. Turn off and let stand for 20 minutes.
2. Beans will plump and bring back to heat and cook again for 40 minutes or until all the water is mostly gone.
3. Or open two cans of Black eye peas and add salt and pepper/ garlic & sautéed onions to taste.

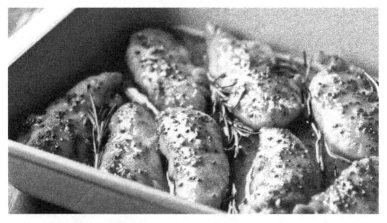

CHICKEN FINGERS IN ROSEMARY SAUCE, PINTO BEANS AND FRENCH FRIED CAULIFLOWER

(For Chicken) Ingredients:

8 to 10 chicken tenders
½ teaspoon of Salt and ground Pepper (or white pepper)
1 teaspoon of ground rosemary powder. Or fresh grounded rosemary excluding stems
1 tablespoon of corn starch

Preparation:

1. Put tenders in a bowl and sprinkle spices and corn starch until covered.
2. Fry in olive oil or canola oil on both sides. Remove from pan and add 1 tablespoon of corn starch and ½ cup of water to pan and

add 1 additional tablespoon of rosemary to the sauce.

3. Replace chicken in the pan and cover both sides of the chicken with the sauce and serve in the sauce.

(Pinto Beans) Preparation:

Cook Pinto beans same as black eye peas or purchase two cans of pinto beans and season to taste with salt and pepper/ garlic and sautéed onions.

(For Cauliflower) Ingredients:

Whole small cauliflower
Flower or bread crumbs
Canola or olive oil
Salt   1 egg
1/3 cup of water

Preparation:

1. Crack open and make egg mixture with egg and salt and water.
2. Cut cauliflower pieces to bite sizes and dip in egg mixture. Then roll into bread crumbs.
3. Prepare a frying pan with canola oil and place the cauliflower in the frying pan and cook on both sides. Or if you have a fryer, drop in fryer and fry like they are French fries. Apply salt when they are finished frying.

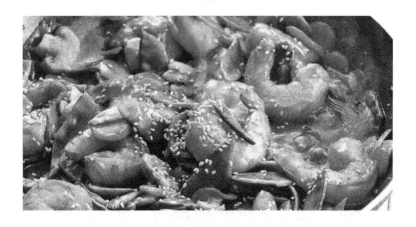

STIR FRIED SHRIMP & VEGETABLES/BOWTIE PASTA

Ingredients:

1 cup of sliced or baby carrots

2 cups of bite size broccoli

1 cup of bite size cauliflower

1 cup of bite sized chopped zucchini

1 tablespoon of Old Bay Seasoning

½ cup of finely chopped parsley

1 Teaspoon of salt/ground pepper

2 cups of 'spring roll' or 'sweet & sour sauce

1 lb. or 3 cups of fresh shrimp cleaned and tail off

For Pasta

1 box of Bow Tie Pasta

½ teaspoon of salt

1 teaspoon of salt and white pepper

Preparation:
1. In a pan of boiling water put the vegetables in the water in the order as listed, Carrots get 2 minutes alone before adding the rest of the vegetable.
2. Cook vegetables until half cooked and remove from the boiling water.
3. In a separate pan, put the vegetables and one cup of sauce together stirring until they obtain the hint of the sauce then add the cooked shrimp and the rest of the sauce.
4. Stir until the mixture is complete with vegetables and shrimp. Serve with Bow tie Pasta,

For Pasta
1. 1 cup of chopped parsley In a pan of boiling water, place the bow tie pasta and season it with I/2 teaspoon of salt.
2. Cook as directed on the box. Drain and add the parsley, salt and white pepper.
3. Stir until all is mixed. A spray of canola oil will help to keep the bow ties separate. Enjoy!

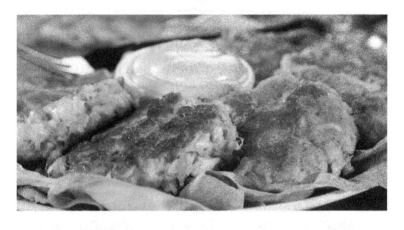

MARYLAND CRAB CAKES & GREEN PEAS AND GOLDEN MASHED POTATOES

(Crab) Ingredients:

I can (1 pound) of crab meat (claws, back fin or special}

2 eggs,

2 cup of bread crumbs

1 tablespoon of mayonnaise

1 1/2 tablespoons of Old Bay Seasoning

1 tablespoon of finely chopped cilantro or parsley

Preparation:

1. Mix crab meat and ingredients together (except for 1 cup of bread crumbs)
2. Make patties and roll the patties in the cup of bread crumbs that is remaining
3. Fry in medium heat in Canola or vegetable oil

until golden brown on both sides

(Green Peas) Ingredients:

Canned or frozen green peas (1 or two depending on diners)
1 teaspoon of salt and pepper.
Cook to desired temperature and taste.

(Potatoes) Ingredients:

Use 6 golden potatoes, not the regular white potatoes as a different starch for this meal
1 tablespoon of salt
1 tablespoon of white pepper
1 quarter cup or 1 half stick of margarine or olive butter

Preparation:

1. Peel, dice, and boil. Strain water and add margarine and salt and white pepper to mashed potatoes.

2. Sprinkle some finely chopped cilantro or parsley in the potatoes.

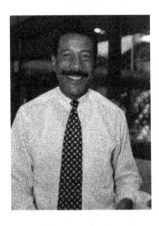

ABOUT THE AUTHOR

David Vaughn is a chef by experience and a caterer by choice. He was born in Baltimore, Maryland, graduated from Morgan State University, Attended Howard University and got an MBA from Pace University in New York City. He worked in Corporate America for almost 30 years. And became a catering Entrepreneur in 1992. His culinary expertise came from a variety of experiences. He is well traveled and he experienced food from Paris, Germany, Egypt, Morocco, Puerto Rico, Brazil and Italy… Not to mention Boston, St. Louis, Chicago, Texas and New Orleans. People say he can cook his butt off, but he doesn't eat everything that he cooks. Why? Because he eats, thinks and does healthy. His philosophy is 'fish, fowl and things that grow.'

-- Hence his reason for creating ideas for healthy living. His first book, "How to Feed Up To 10 People for under $10," was well publicized in Essence, Black Enterprise and The Baltimore Sun in 1982 Many years before he started his new life style… A Healthier Life."

David is available for workshops, seminars, and other speaking engagements. To book David for your next event, please email him at dvaughn101@comcast.net.

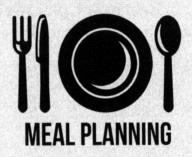

MEAL PLANNING

GOAL TRACKER FOR THE MONTH OF _____

ORGANIZATION

CLEANING

PLANNING

BUDGET

MEAL PLAN

EXERCISE

WEEK 1 WATER ●●●●●●●●
EXERCISE ☐☐☐☐☐☐☐☐

WEEK 1 WATER ●●●●●●●●
EXERCISE ☐☐☐☐☐☐☐☐

WEEK 1 WATER ●●●●●●●●
EXERCISE ☐☐☐☐☐☐☐☐

WEEK 1 WATER ●●●●●●●●
EXERCISE ☐☐☐☐☐☐☐☐

MEAL PLAN

STARTING _____

ENDING _____

GOAL TRACKER FOR THE MONTH OF _____

ORGANIZATION

CLEANING

PLANNING

BUDGET

MEAL PLAN

EXERCISE

WEEK 1 WATER ●●●●●●● EXERCISE ☐☐☐☐☐☐☐☐

WEEK 1 WATER ●●●●●●●● EXERCISE ☐☐☐☐☐☐☐☐

WEEK 1 WATER ●●●●●●●● EXERCISE ☐☐☐☐☐☐☐☐

WEEK 1 WATER ●●●●●●●● EXERCISE ☐☐☐☐☐☐☐☐

MEAL PLAN

STARTING _____

ENDING _____

GROCERY LIST _____

FRUITS	ITEM	QTY

MEAT	ITEM	QTY

DAIRY	ITEM	QTY

VEGETABLES	ITEM	QTY

GROCERY LIST

	ITEM	QTY
DAIRY		

	ITEM	QTY
PASTA/RICE		

	ITEM	QTY
CEREAL		

	ITEM	QTY
SNACKS		

WEEKLY PLANNED MEALS _____

BREAKFAST						
SNACK						
LUNCH						
SNACK						
DINNER						
SNACK						

WEEKLY PLANNED MEALS _____

BREAKFAST						
SNACK						
LUNCH						
SNACK						
DINNER						
SNACK						

WEEKLY PLANNED MEALS _____

	S	M	T	W	T	F	S
BREAKFAST							
SNACK							
LUNCH							
SNACK							
DINNER							
SNACK							

WEEKLY PLANNED MEALS _____

BREAKFAST							
SNACK							
LUNCH							
SNACK							
DINNER							
SNACK							

WEEKLY PLANNED MEALS _____

BREAKFAST							
SNACK							
LUNCH							
SNACK							
DINNER							
SNACK							

WEEKLY PLANNED MEALS _____

BREAKFAST							
SNACK							
LUNCH							
SNACK							
DINNER							
SNACK							

WEEKLY PLANNED MEALS _____

BREAKFAST						
SNACK						
LUNCH						
SNACK						
DINNER						
SNACK						

WEEKLY PLANNED MEALS _____

BREAKFAST							
SNACK							
LUNCH							
SNACK							
DINNER							
SNACK							

WEEKLY PLANNED MEALS _____

	S	M	T	W	T	F	S
BREAKFAST							
SNACK							
LUNCH							
SNACK							
DINNER							
SNACK							

WEEKLY PLANNED MEALS _____

BREAKFAST							
SNACK							
LUNCH							
SNACK							
DINNER							
SNACK							

WEEKLY PLANNED MEALS _____

BREAKFAST						
SNACK						
LUNCH						
SNACK						
DINNER						
SNACK						

WEEKLY PLANNED MEALS _____

	S	M	T	W	T	F	S
BREAKFAST							
SNACK							
LUNCH							
SNACK							
DINNER							
SNACK							

WEEKLY PLANNED MEALS _____

	S	M	T	W	T	F	S
BREAKFAST							
SNACK							
LUNCH							
SNACK							
DINNER							
SNACK							

MONTHLY MEAL PLANNER FOR _____

WEEK 1						
WEEK 2						
WEEK 3						
WEEK 4						
WEEK 5						
WEEK 6						

MONTHLY MEAL PLANNER FOR _____

	S	M	T	W	T	F	S
WEEK 1	☐	☐	☐	☐	☐	☐	☐
WEEK 2	☐	☐	☐	☐	☐	☐	☐
WEEK 3	☐	☐	☐	☐	☐	☐	☐
WEEK 4	☐	☐	☐	☐	☐	☐	☐
WEEK 5	☐	☐	☐	☐	☐	☐	☐
WEEK 6	☐	☐	☐	☐	☐	☐	☐

MONTHLY MEAL PLANNER FOR _____

	S	M	T	W	T	F	S
WEEK 1	☐	☐	☐	☐	☐	☐	☐
WEEK 2	☐	☐	☐	☐	☐	☐	☐
WEEK 3	☐	☐	☐	☐	☐	☐	☐
WEEK 4	☐	☐	☐	☐	☐	☐	☐
WEEK 5	☐	☐	☐	☐	☐	☐	☐
WEEK 6	☐	☐	☐	☐	☐	☐	☐

MONTHLY MEAL PLANNER FOR _____

	S	M	T	W	T	F	S
WEEK 1	☐	☐	☐	☐	☐	☐	☐
WEEK 2	☐	☐	☐	☐	☐	☐	☐
WEEK 3	☐	☐	☐	☐	☐	☐	☐
WEEK 4	☐	☐	☐	☐	☐	☐	☐
WEEK 5	☐	☐	☐	☐	☐	☐	☐
WEEK 6	☐	☐	☐	☐	☐	☐	☐

MONTHLY MEAL PLANNER FOR _____

WEEK 1	☐	☐	☐	☐	☐	☐	☐
WEEK 2	☐	☐	☐	☐	☐	☐	☐
WEEK 3	☐	☐	☐	☐	☐	☐	☐
WEEK 4	☐	☐	☐	☐	☐	☐	☐
WEEK 5	☐	☐	☐	☐	☐	☐	☐
WEEK 6	☐	☐	☐	☐	☐	☐	☐

MONTHLY MEAL PLANNER FOR _____

WEEK 1	☐	☐	☐	☐	☐	☐	☐
WEEK 2	☐	☐	☐	☐	☐	☐	☐
WEEK 3	☐	☐	☐	☐	☐	☐	☐
WEEK 4	☐	☐	☐	☐	☐	☐	☐
WEEK 5	☐	☐	☐	☐	☐	☐	☐
WEEK 6	☐	☐	☐	☐	☐	☐	☐

MONTHLY MEAL PLANNER FOR _____

WEEK 1

WEEK 2

WEEK 3

WEEK 4

WEEK 5

WEEK 6

MONTHLY MEAL PLANNER FOR _____

	S	M	T	W	T	F	S
WEEK 1	☐	☐	☐	☐	☐	☐	☐
WEEK 2	☐	☐	☐	☐	☐	☐	☐
WEEK 3	☐	☐	☐	☐	☐	☐	☐
WEEK 4	☐	☐	☐	☐	☐	☐	☐
WEEK 5	☐	☐	☐	☐	☐	☐	☐
WEEK 6	☐	☐	☐	☐	☐	☐	☐

MONTHLY MEAL PLANNER FOR _____

WEEK 1 ☐	☐	☐	☐	☐	☐	☐
WEEK 2 ☐	☐	☐	☐	☐	☐	☐
WEEK 3 ☐	☐	☐	☐	☐	☐	☐
WEEK 4 ☐	☐	☐	☐	☐	☐	☐
WEEK 5 ☐	☐	☐	☐	☐	☐	☐
WEEK 6 ☐	☐	☐	☐	☐	☐	☐

MONTHLY MEAL PLANNER FOR _____

WEEK 1	☐	☐	☐	☐	☐	☐	☐
WEEK 2	☐	☐	☐	☐	☐	☐	☐
WEEK 3	☐	☐	☐	☐	☐	☐	☐
WEEK 4	☐	☐	☐	☐	☐	☐	☐
WEEK 5	☐	☐	☐	☐	☐	☐	☐
WEEK 6	☐	☐	☐	☐	☐	☐	☐

MONTHLY MEAL PLANNER FOR _____

WEEK 1	☐	☐	☐	☐	☐	☐
WEEK 2	☐	☐	☐	☐	☐	☐
WEEK 3	☐	☐	☐	☐	☐	☐
WEEK 4	☐	☐	☐	☐	☐	☐
WEEK 5	☐	☐	☐	☐	☐	☐
WEEK 6	☐	☐	☐	☐	☐	☐

CPSIA information can be obtained
at www.ICGtesting.com
Printed in the USA
FSHW01n0827300518
48611FS